P9-DTF-275

DATE DUE

DE 16 97			
NY 6			

DEMCO 38-296

HOW NOT
TO CATCH
A COLD

A sure effective guide
for passing through cold
seasons without catching cold.

Riverside Community College
Library
4800 Magnolia Avenue
Riverside, California 92506

HOW NOT TO CATCH A COLD

H. Dehesh

GP

GLOBAL PUBLISHING

Riverside Community College
Library
4800 Magnolia Avenue
Riverside, California 92506

© 1991 by H. Dehesh.

RF 361 .D44 1996

Dehesh, Hadayat, 1924-

How not to catch a cold   ehesh.

          1. Cold (Disease)—Prevention—Popular works. I.
     Title.
     RF361.D44 1995   616.2′05′05
                                            QBI95-20663

Global Publishing
17352 W. 12 Mile Rd, Suite 201
Southfield, MI 48076

When I Catch the Cold
I don't feel so bold.
Courage! Are you too
Affected by the cold?

To Hell With All New Medicine
I Hunger bad, for Going back
To What is Good and Old.

To

my daughter HEDYEH

Contents

Chapter I

Dear Tammy,

As you know by now I returned to the U.S. after not having been there for more than a decade. I came for my daughter's graduation, and thought I would stop in New York and see you before my flight back to Europe and then, Iran.

In your wonderful city, where most of the population lives in the stratosphere with only service connections to earth, I had the loneliest time, living in a hotel room, way up and up, waiting for a telephone call that never came. I called your office, and your secretary told me that you would not be in for a few days.

After some preliminary probing on her part and mine, and my telling her I was an old friend from the university days, she told me that you were home, down with a cold. Her tone, while polite, intimated that the conversation should end there and this reminded me of your house-mother in Berkeley. (History was repeating itself once more.)

So many times when we were students, that hopeless news derailed my expectation for a chat with you on the phone, a ride around the green hills, a movie, a walk, dinner, studying together at the library, a snack before ten—so many things—that my memory is unable to recount them all now. The visitation of the cold virus with you was nearly once every three months, as I remember, and now with the passage of so many years confession comes easy:

In those days, at times, a sickening worry overwhelmed me when I was told you couldn't come to the phone because of a bout with the cold. I always thought it was a ploy, a prelude to avoid seeing a foreign student who forever was confused about the big question: to be or not to be in America after graduation. Your voice, hoarse from the cold, when days later you spoke to me on the phone sounded to my ear better than nightingales singing. It had a steadying effect always, restored my sense of confidence, and made me feel like a prince.

It was my wanting to hear your voice again this time, hoarse or not, that I hustled verbally with your secretary a while more than she had patience for, but she just wouldn't come through with your home phone number. Since I knew beforehand that you were unlisted, your secretary was the only line of hope, but she was firm and noncommittal.

Finally, I made her note my full difficult name, my hotel and room number. As assertively as I could, I told her to convey the message that I was expecting your return call at the earliest. With condescending coolness she said that she would convey the message, in the event you call the office. She was not one to be thrown so easily, but I had a mind to tell her a few things. Sorry, Tammy, I was about to snap out that I had partially financed the business in which she now worked and earned a salary, but a thought flashed in my mind on time. I braked.

After an instant of silence I said goodbye.

With a good-riddance drawl just like your house-mother she said, "You are welcome," which to me sounded like a despairing curse.

About the money I loaned you and you paid back in full with a token interest, let me tell you that was the only money I had transferred out of the country before the Revolution. In my heyday before the great upheaval, golden opportunities were overlooked in this respect because I was one of those second-rate thinkers, who thought the regime of the Shah would last and that Iran was a bastion of security in the Middle East. All underlying indications were otherwise, but they didn't register on me. Even at the peak of the uprising, I didn't believe the regime was gasping its last dying breath.

I held on tight in the squalling storm, became in no time, like many others, a goner with the wind. I found and lost, same as the case was between you and me.

But you well know I am not a cantankerous loser. I scrambled up the rocks again, quietly, reached a scale not as high as before but near it. I admit, during those early hard years after the

Revolution, without that money in your hand I would not have been able to send my son through college. He is my double now, a full-fledged mechanical engineer working with me. So, a quirk of fate reversed things. I became indebted to you. This was the thought that flashed in my mind in time and stopped me from losing my head with your secretary.

Having been unsuccessful with her, I stood for quite a while by the window of my hotel room watching the immense, manmade skyline of Manhattan. Swift memories of the past came to me. Gradually the morose mood in me changed as I remembered the times we had together.

I recalled once how you and I, after class, went together to the university hospital and had our tonsils painted—the only remedy available at the time for sore throats.

Now with my mind's eye I saw you in a spacious bedroom, alone, a large glass of water standing by your bedside, surrounded with huge capsules of red, brown, yellow and blue. Your winsome face, pale and weary, devoid of the make-up of the fashion world, grimaced repeatedly for an expected sneeze that sometimes refused to come. A plastic basket full of used tissue paper sat by your bedside on the floor.

Fired up with the knowledge that I could help you, in more ways than the one hundred thousand I loaned you, I felt in me the audacity of Cary Grant in "Notorious": walking up the curved stairway with elegance overshadowing stealth to save a doped and dazed Ingrid Bergman from the programmed poisoning of Nazi conspirators in Argentine. The picture ended with him daringly saving Ingrid. We saw that picture together when it first came out. Remember? If I knew the place of your residence I would have walked up, ignoring the severe threats and protestation of your maid.

Your secretary, standing at the top of the stairway, would stare down at me with curled lips as I walked up. I would enter your bedroom and sit by your bedside. Your wan face would turn, brightening slowly with a smile of recognition, and soon our hands would hold in perfect strength like old times in the movies.

❧

Seeing you concerned about my catching your cold—which as before I never cared about—I would start telling you, Tammy, about my not having bouts with a cold for more than ten years, not in the usual, accepted sense. Like most people you wouldn't believe me at first. I could read your thoughts: how could I have discovered something about the sure-cure of influenza when the medical researchers in this field hadn't. It is said that in tight spots one becomes an inventor. I have been in many a tight spot with a cold and I hated it. I hated it so much that I preferred to have a bout with tuberculosis once in a lifetime than have a soul-sickening bout with a cold once or twice every year.

For more than ten years, a time stretch that doesn't leave grounds for doubts, I haven't gone to bed with a cold and then come out debilitated, looking like the Phantom of Opera.

I haven't lost a single day of work or activity in the last ten years. Even the flu epidemics of the past years with their menacing Asiatic names like Hong Kong flu, Chinese, Burmese, Shanghai, Taiwan, Yamagata and so on, have not been able to de-capacitate me.

I have learned how to combat the virus effectively. I have licked the problem totally and completely. I wouldn't bat an eye if I hear that this year's virus is the meanest and it comes from Madagascar or wherever, but for inquiry's sake, why is it that a cold virus never comes from Europe? Why don't we ever hear a Cote de'Azure flu or Manchester flu.

The World Health Organization is responsible for explaining this phenomenon, but the East is East and the West is West and on a rare occasion when the two meet, we do get a word like influenza, which is a corruption of the Arabic word "anf-al-anza." "Anf" in Arabic means nose and "al-anza" means the goat. A coughing, drooling, nose-dripping goat is said to have "anfalanza"—goatnosed—which could apply easily to a human in the same condition. The *American Heritage Dictionary* specifies the Latin word "influentia," meaning "influence," as the origin of the word "influenza," but that doesn't make sense. Disclaiming erudition, "anfalanza" is more apt to

♥

be the origin of the word in my opinion. The goatnosed condition applies more firmly and more believably.

Deeply floundering in the morbidity of a bad cold some people, not consciously knowing the connection, say, "I feel like a sick goat." Now if the outbreak-source and name of the disease is from the East, so let the cure come from the East also, however unorthodox, as always, it may seem to those who are not from the East.

First things first, Tammy, there must be a total change in attitude toward a cold, in regard to the range of it, whether it is bacterial or viral. The acceptance that there is no such thing as a minor cold, that all colds become major ones—especially the flu version—when you refuse to rest, is a great understanding of the problem, but greater still is the acceptance of the fact that rest, when the early signs of a cold come, is a theory cure and is quite impossible.

You just cannot jump headlong into bed and start a two-day's rest because your throat tickles or you blew your nose twice before breakfast. A normally active person just cannot idle himself like that.

All those who go to bed with a cold are those who have reached such a stage of incapacity that they have no choice, or they are exceptional people who can stop the impetus of life in themselves with the ease of one turning off a switch. These people are much less than a minority. On a mass scale, forced rest as a preventive measure could never be brought about.

Either you have an important appointment that cannot be canceled, a job of some kind that must be finished, a deadline that must be met, a report on a project that must be completed, or you will not have much of a life. The inertial force cannot easily be stopped.

In the meantime the intruding virus breeds and multiplies. You become weak. Your ears plug from too much nose-blowing, your head pounds, and your eyes water. Gradually the world becomes meaningless to you. You go to bed finally, sick. All prescribed or recommended medicines for a cold at this stage are palliatives which make life only easier while the sickness runs its course.

❦

After you get well, excluding the after-effects there is a period of immunity—during which you won't catch a cold ranging three months in your case, six in mine in the old days and with most people a full year.

My formula rests on the theory that if any kind or version of a cold virus gives you immunity for a certain period after the sickness, why not reduce the initial invading virus to a level of weakness that it becomes a vaccine against itself and all other similar cold viruses to which you may be exposed?

How can this be done? The magic is in combat readiness, and this requires a singular passion to overcome an epidemic to which the world has been accustomed, accepting its terms year after year, unconditionally. You must develop the old cowboy mentality of the western movies. After a long ride during the day, the cowboy sleeps in the woods by the fire with his head on the saddle and his trigger-finger on his gun. When his horse snorts signaling danger, he jumps, ready for a quick shoot-out.

At the first sign of being stricken with a cold,

strike back hard and quick. Don't take it lying down. Don't lose precious hours finding out whether the tickle in your throat, the wretched chill or the mildly running nose is going to go away by itself. Experience repeatedly has proven that it will not, but we always tend to think otherwise.

Every year we lull ourselves with a perfidious optimism expecting a miracle cure, that the deceptively mild cold on the onset will let go, but it doesn't. The virus overwhelms. That is one thing we can be sure of.

As the clock ticks on, an empty bed is there to embrace you when you don't want its embrace. The demon virus brings depression and a lassitude so grave you may feel at times that you will never get well, will never become whole again. The old confident self becomes remote.

In the old days, citrus juice was an accepted requirement for cold patients because of its vitamin C content. Science has now fully approved the old notion that this worthy vitamin is the one and only combatant known that can lock horns with the mean, circular, face-and-trait changing cold virus. Thus, as part of your battle readiness, have a bottle of vitamin C (ascorbic acid) in tablets of 500 mg strength in your medicine cabinet, but don't take a daily dose when you are well and healthy.

Taking a daily dose of vitamin C as preventive medicine is like shooting wildly every day into the sky with the hopes that a duck will fall at your feet. The effect of vitamin C taken orally is not cumulative. The tablets taken on the day or day before exposure to the virus are helpful— not those you took four months ago. Besides, taking vitamin C tablets as part of the daily diet increases your saliva to a point that you have to swallow first before you can talk.

Just have the vitamin C tablets in your medicine cabinet for the D-day, and don't drink either orange or grapefruit juice daily to a level that keeps you on the verge of diarrhea. Lead a normal life. Don't get edgy when you come into contact with people who have a cold, and don't resort to bizarre behavior in order to avoid them.

If the catching of a cold can be useful as a mild vaccination of a cold, why not catch it earlier? The more advanced in autumn, or late summer, the least is the after-effect. Therefore, when someone sneezes helplessly in an elevator or subway or any other closed space, don't flinch grievously in order to shame him.

Even if you lived under a glass bell, the catching of a cold is certain when the season for it comes. Most often you are the carrier of the virus without being affected. The intrusion takes place when your resistance is lowered by either exposure to cold, fatigue, hunger or even anger for a long period of time. Depression also welcomes the catching of a cold. (I will come back to that with more details.)

Now let us say that the virus has invaded and the early signs are there: sneezing, the consistent wet nose and a chill while the thermometer on the wall shows eighty. Move fast. Remember that you are not going to take it from the virus anymore. You are prepared for a quick counterattack, even if the time is most inconvenient, say, you have guests in the house for the evening.

Excuse yourself for a while. Go to the bathroom, and close the door—you don't want advice or interruption. Drop a 500-mg vitamin C tablet into a drinking glass, and tap it with something blunt, like the butt end of a knife until it is in powder form. You can use powdered vitamin C with the same dosage about 500 mg. Add about two shot glasses of water. Stir. Be prepared for the most unorthodox and excruciating part of the treatment, and remember that anything not done on a mass scale appears odd.

Once upon a time the simple act of an injection with a needle looked odd and excruciatingly painful to the onlookers as well as the patient, but we are all now much accustomed to it.

Pour the VC solution into your cupped hand and draw it up into your nostrils, your nasal passage, and throat, then spit out the excrement. Repeat this procedure three or four times. The solution in the glass should be finished if you have the right concentration. When you do this you will gag, Tammy, with a burning ache that peaks out in twenty seconds after that last draw.

During the takes, you cough, sniffle and snort, and a thick liquid will come down from your nasal passages in mouthfuls, and you will blow your nose and spit out repeatedly. This gelatin-like goo, dislodged so devastatingly, happens to be the bedding where the virus proliferates. And you will wonder how and where in the small narrow passage so much of it could be stored.

Using the strongest word, your suffering, for this treatment is less than a minute, nowhere comparable to what you have to bear if you let the cold go into full blooming growth.

With the vitamin C wash, you decimate the virus and destroy its breeding haven. This bold act gives you time for the next move. The virus, too, takes a new position, increases in number, but not with as much force and spirit as before. You have brought havoc into the routine of the virus. Their situation after the VC wash is like the setting of camps on the rubble after an earthquake.

You, however, come out of the bathroom breathing like a giant. Your nasal passages are open, clear, and free. Air flows into your lungs, and comes with such ease that it is as if your nostrils and the passages beyond them have the inner diameter of a four-inch pipe. You become suffused with a state of well-being, though for a while you might look as if you had wept.

Sometimes with this simple inexpensive act, you will succeed in flushing the cold virus out of your system, but most often, especially if it is an autumn cold, you will not. Take a sleeping pill or any kind of sedative that night and go to bed early. You have further treatment coming the next day.

Chapter II

Now, Tammy, don't think that what I have prescribed so far is a frightful thing. Don't seek the counsel of friends and doctors. Don't wait for the Surgeon General to approve this. Just be bold enough to do it once and see the magic results, and don't think that if you draw the solution of vitamin C repeatedly into your nose you are going to end up with your nose gone. Ascorbic acid is just not that kind of acid.

I have snorted in a VC solution at least two times a year for the past years, and the great masterpiece of a nose that I have is still there, ever keen of the sense of smell and ever filtering the heavily polluted air of Tehran for my durable lungs.

I have tried a weaker solution on my young

daughter who now is four and a half years old. Whenever she has a running nose, I let her have it with an eye-dropper. When I hear her soft breathing while she is asleep, I know that the magic wash was of great service to her, in spite of her screaming which she would do anyway even if the drops were water.

Only when she is running a fever do I take her to a doctor. For simple colds I give her the VC wash, and VC sherbet made out of a VC tablet in powdered form with water and sugar, which she drinks with more relish than orange juice or soda pop.

There are many nose drops available that open plugged noses, but their effect is temporary. You have to repeat the drops after a couple of hours. You do this only once with the VC wash, for which there is absolutely no substitute when you are in the clutches of a cold. You can repeat-wash once every eight hours if you want and do nothing else, but this would be like hit-and-run warfare with the virus. There is no need for it. We have the means of delivering the enemy one quick mortal blow the morning after.

❦

After a restful night's sleep, you wake up re-
freshed. As soon as you begin preparing for the
day, the symptoms of a cold on the make appear
again. The virus brood wasn't idle while you were
sleeping. Among your home-stored medicine you
must keep two ampules of 500 mg vitamin C for
intravenous injection and one dose of gamma
globulin. Keep these in the refrigerator. Take one
of each and go to a clinic, a professional nurse,
the family doctor or an injection center (not
available in your country), whichever is more
readily available to you.

Have an intravenous injection of the vitamin
C and then, in the same session, a hip shot of the
gamma globulin. Do this at least once. I will be
gratified that my writing you this letter is not a
vain effort.

By the time you pull up your pants—if you
happen to be wearing one, Tammy—you will no
longer be afflicted with a curse-deserving cold. If
it is not Saturday, Sunday or a holiday, go to
work, attend to your business in full, and don't
worry about your cold becoming worse. Con-

sider yourself vaccinated and accept the lethargy, which comes after any vaccination.

When the night comes, go to bed early and take a sedative, not necessarily to induce an early sleep, but for unwinding totally and giving your sleep depth when it comes. Sleep speeds recovery, drug-induced or not, from any illness. Sedative taking is the secret of one getting well much quicker in a hospital. In all hospitals the night nurse always comes a couple of hours after dinner with a small plastic cup with several sleep-related pills for every patient. They even wake up a sleeping patient and give him sleeping pills. Have not qualms about taking pills to induce sleep when ill, but avoid dependence on them when you are well.

The next day, if the cold is still with you, even mildly, deliver it the *coup de grace*: another intravenous shot of vitamin C. After that go play eighteen holes of golf if you want to, attend your dancing, aerobic, gymnastic or yoga class, but get your sleep and avoid eating or drinking anything outright from the refrigerator.

From this point on until the end of the winter, if you happen to be wearing light clothes not suitable for a cold day, you will only feel cold. The wretched chill doesn't come with exposure to cold temperatures or exposure to a virus from others. You can go to the sauna, come out and drop yourself in the snow if your heart is stout enough to take the shock. I do that sometimes, after having sat with people in the sauna who foolishly have come there to get rid of their "damn" cold.

Some people also think they can knock their *damned* cold out with alcohol. They get crocked or they imbibe a warm concoction with either rum, cognac or whiskey (in Iran homemade vodka) as its base. Useless. During a bout with a cold, and days after, the only alcohol good for you is the amount in a cough syrup, and that is not enough to keep your windpipe warm for long.

Individual experimentation with a gimmick cure shall prevail but there is an absolute, unmistakable cure in the available medicine and the gimmick lies only on lightning-speed application. Gamma globulin or flu shots have been recommended as a preventive measure prior to catching a cold, but it is difficult to induce good and healthy people to inject themselves when the exigencies of an illness doesn't exist.

Besides, the effectiveness of gamma globulin fades with time, and it is unlikely that you would know or remember the complete fade-out time. You catch a cold, perhaps a milder one, just like having had flu shots, but you have to live with a cold again until it is over, which is the same and not at all acceptable to me. But with this proposed formula, based on a quick response with gamma globulin, which is most potent on delivery, and vitamin C from an in-shot and out-wash, you only notice and bear for a short time the symptoms of a cold and never a full-fledged cold, never the flu itself.

If the suggested plan at first glance seems elaborate, fortify your will by thinking about the indignity of feeling the wetness of a saturated handkerchief in your trouser's pocket.

The mass-media has hammered into our heads year after year that there is no cure for a common cold, that we have to live with it as an accepted fate with the costs running into billions of dollars annually in lost productivity. I bet you anything, Tammy, you and your forty employees can prove the mass-media wrong and the mass-despondency unjustified.

Absenteeism in schools and industry because of catching colds could be reduced drastically. Suffering from influenza, too, could become a thing of the past. If there is a will there is a way.

Execute the method on yourself at the outbreak of a cold, if it is your lot to be infected before most others. Then with reliance on personal knowledge, gather your employees and deliver a speech. Tell them first what they must know. Tell them that things have gotten so out of hand that you just can't take it from the virus anymore. Insist on their having those inexpensive medicines ready at home, and you have them also available at the office. Forty employees incapacitated, on the average, three days a year is equivalent to one employee's absence because of ill health, one hundred and twenty days a year. Transpose this on 100 million working people in the U.S. alone and see the astonishing cost of absenteeism.

You and your organization, tell them, are just not going to take that anymore. When one of your fitters sneezes with a quick-dispelling mist spewing before his or her face, get set for delivery of the full treatment. The VC wash first. If you have a cooperative professional nurse at phone's-reach, call. After she arrives, the whole thing doesn't take five minutes—the vitamin C and the gamma globulin shots.

I don't believe that among the entire working population in the world there is one who prefers being sick in bed with a cold, than working.

After you have treated yourself only once, and you come forth talking with the acquired faith and knowledge that the treatment is failproof, you will meet only the full cooperation of your employees. With full confidence you can tell your audience that the flu shots recommended as the best protection against a cold are only second best to what you prescribe. The method of quick response and decimating the number and strength of the attacking viruses in your body, regardless of strain or origin, is the best method.

The flu shots available this year are made from the strain of the previous year's virus, cultivated in egg embryos. The vaccine produces antibodies for the strain of the virus that spread the previous year. Now, if the strain this year is different from last year, the flu shots are not quite effective. The virus, in medical language, is said to mutate, changing chemical profile and personality once every two to three years and there are strains A, B and C. When the host population becomes immune to one strain, the virus changes structure.

So who knows what exactly is coming next year? Which pharmaceutical company could produce the exact, right-on-the-nail flu shot for the year to come? The enemy is devious and clever.

The enemy is mean, too, and the flu shots cannot prevent the invasion, cannot prevent an epidemic. Epidemics can only be prevented by individual effort on a mass scale with the no nonsense theory of quicker than quick response.

Besides, can everyone afford the flu shot price: twenty-five dollars a shot, or more, for one person? Can a family on welfare afford that? A nose wash with vitamin C solution costs a few cents and if you can bear the discomfort, the repeat-wash during a cold is as good as a flu shot. It brings the cold to a level of a mild one, which is what the flu shot does.

There are doubts about the effectiveness of the flu shots in the medical profession also. Under the heading "Doubts Over Influenza Vaccine—Does Mass Use Do Any Good?" *Medical News* reported that "three senior U.S. Public Health Service doctors expressed doubts about the value of mass influenza immunization programs. Their case rests upon the fact that excess deaths from influenza and pneumonia reached a figure of 12,000 during last February and March and April, despite 42 million doses of influenza vaccine used." This was reported on November 22, 1963, but with 8100 flu-related deaths in the U.S. in the past and current year, I don't believe conditions have improved any. So heed my letter carefully, Tammy.

Gamma globulin and vitamin C ampules are not drug counter medicines. But until the right law is enacted, you have to get it like people who got moonshine during Prohibition.

For the time being, a friendly pharmacist can help. A year's supply is only two ampules per adult, which unfortunately for a normal person is harder to get than an addict obtaining his daily supply of heroin, cocaine or crack in the streets of New York.

The medical profession must make it easy for those who want these ampules. They should be willing to prescribe them to healthy, reliable people for safekeeping in their medicine cabinets. The Food and Drug Administration should even allow the sale of these harmless medicines without a doctor's prescription.

A flu epidemic begins abruptly and reaches a peak within two to three weeks. How can millions of patients be treated in such a sudden eruption? When doctor offices become overloaded, their home and office phones keep ringing and hospital beds become scarce, it can hardly be said that because of *anfalanza* they are having their finest hour. They should relinquish the early treatment to people themselves, since people can not reach them early enough. Besides, what can doctors do except mainly recommend rest when the cold is at an advanced stage?

Injection centers must be set up throughout the country, or better, people should be trained to inoculate themselves, like diabetics do. A wife or a husband trained to give VC and GG shots could save the whole family, and if this becomes common practice the wind could be knocked out of any viral epidemic no matter how bad it would be otherwise.

Intravenous shots require extensive training. A clumsy injectionist could sieve one arm before the needle finds its way into the vein. And if he injects a drop outside the vein it would be very painful.

If the VC shot is going to be delivered by a non-medic, best it be delivered in the hip. Unfortunately, you walk around feeling like you have a piece of acid-soaked lead deep inside your buttocks for a period lasting about two hours. The more you walk the quicker it gets absorbed in the blood. The pain fades. The advantage of the intravenous shot is that you only feel the insertion of the needle at the start, and that is all.

Of course there will be mishaps and abuses. A woman might do away with an unwanted husband with a non-detectable agent mixed with the injection of vitamin C or gamma globulin, either to hasten an inheritance or just for good riddance. A few might experience shock or some unforeseen after-effects. Allergies must also be kept in mind.

But what is all this compared to all the benefits? Could car accidents ever outweigh the benefit of cars? We would never kill, maim or permanently disable each other if we all walked, but society would stop functioning if cars stopped moving on the roads.

We should refrain from harping on imagined, isolated tragedies that may occur. If ordinary people went to injection classes and just learned how to inoculate themselves and each other, we would not and could not have epidemics, but would suffer only isolated cases of the illness. No longer would we see billions of dollars lost in productivity every year.

❦

For years to come this condition will not change unless we change our attitude toward the catching of colds. We should not deliver our beings like sacrificial lambs to the virus every year as an accepted fate.

When the virus invades and person-to-person transmission starts, there really is no stopping it. If near half the population of a city comes down with the virus and they have faith in the quick response, and if they request injections of vitamin C and gamma globulin, there will not be enough doctors and professional nurses to balance the immense need. And if there be any long waiting in the corridors of a hospital or in the home of a nurse, the concept of quick response shall be lost, which is the most important thing.

The washing of your nasal passages with the vitamin C solution is for the purpose of giving you time. But this time is limited. You have to move fast with the injection of the recommended ampules. If the population acquires faith in the method, there will not be enough doctors or professional nurses to meet the demand. The best choice, therefore, is to have at least one member of the family attend class in a clinic and receive an injection certificate.

If all medications pertaining to catching a cold are to remain under the supervision of the medical profession, one could, with a wild Twilight-Zone-type imagination, envision assembly lines set up in hospitals with robots injecting vitamin C and gamma globulin in patients lying with bare behinds, cheeks up, on a conveyor belt.

The woman's section comes to mind first. Just think—derrieres of different shapes and colors, flaccid or robust, huge or puny, moving irreversibly toward two bright, shining needles. The robot injects each with electronic precision at the right spot with the right dose of vitamin C and gamma globulin. The used needles get discarded by compressed air and new ones are picked up by vacuum. With their heads resting on the backs of their hands, the women will chat amicably about fashion, health-food, calorie intake, husbands, and all sorts of other subjects, as theirs comes inexorably beneath the needles.

This would be in sharp contrast with the

penal machine in Kafka's *Penal Colony*, where the prisoner's sentence written by needles on his flesh speeded up the penetration of guilt into his consciousness for the good of the state.

It would be good if the world, as predicted, reaches the end of history. The Orwellian vision of the future is fading fast: 1984 has passed. Governments gushing forth with slogans are giving way to governments of reason. Mass deception is becoming ever more intangible. There will be no more world wars, no more gulags or penal colonies, and no more inventions of more efficient torture machines.

In a decaying world man's greatest enemy shall be the virus. AIDS is the front runner. AIDS and environmental decay together will make history—the two came on in the same era and one cannot escape the mental association. With a ruptured ozone layer our good-ship-lollipop earth seems to have lost its virginity, as well as its innocence, all from the inside.

Chapter III

I guess, Tammy, if you ever run for political office you would never make me your speech writer. But what else can one think of except assembly line medication when tens of millions are in the grip of the virus, or are about to receive its visitation and fall flat in bed weary and depressed.

The virus is so highly contagious that you can't fend it off unless you are fully prepared. One sneeze by a passenger in an airplane and—bing!—the virus has found a home but not necessarily the soil to proliferate. You get it, even though you are sitting fifty feet away from the passenger who sneezed. The air in the airplane is recirculated, and it would have made no difference if the passenger had let it go with a sneeze right into your face.

Even on the ground in a closed space with people sitting in an air-conditioned area, which as a rule re-circulates seventy-five percent of the inlet air, there really is no escape from that person who has this temporary disease sitting anywhere in that closed space. You're at risk even in a theater or a movie. These circumstances make you catch colds, reasons can be imagined or to be remained unknown.

After forty-eight hours or so, if you are prone, the classic symptoms including a running nose, headache, muscle aches and sometimes sore throat come, and you always think you had made some mistake like sitting in a draft or not having your jacket on while watering the lawn.

From 412 B.C. on, when a viral disease was described by the Greek physician Hippocrates, man has borne the viral infection with a considerable measure of self-blame and unjustified guilt. Exposure to low temperature only speeds the onset of the infection. That is all it does.

The assembly line concept can wait until it is desperately needed. For now the individual effort will do and there is no shortness of anything to achieve invincibility.

And you know, for some reason, by fighting the cold virus year after year and on time with the method described, in regard to your resistance, you mutate into a different being. A metamorphosis takes place.

When you don't fear the cold virus and you are prepared to welcome it any time, you seem to develop the type of antibody that makes you immune to catching the strain of virus that brings headaches, muscle aches and fever. It is always the wet-nose type that comes, year after year, which doesn't get anywhere with anyone exercising the method.

I have even better news for you, Tammy, coming at the end of this letter. So read on.

Regarding a sore throat, age must have some influence, but I haven't been bothered with one in the last ten years. There have been times I had a peculiar sensation in my throat when swallowing, but it has been so minor that I have either gargled with salt water or just ignored it.

I believe if the method I've described above is

exercised by the whole population of the earth, the breeding ground for the virus will become so inhospitable that eventually the virus will die out, will be exterminated, just like smallpox. But for that to happen, all this scaremongering that you should not take a pill or any medicine without consulting a physician out of the fear of harming yourself must end.

There are minor illnesses with their cure within the range, scope and knowledge of many adults, because of their past experiences with the illness. Only they don't dare to do anything on their own because of all the fear that only doctors should recommend the right medicine.

In regard to influenza there is great confusion. There are countless theories, hypotheses and contradictions among the medical community. While residing in the U.S., I was once given penicillin shots by a doctor for influenza. Not that it did me any good at all, but another doctor, on hearing this, shook his head and conveyed with his fixed gaze that the other doctor, whom he didn't know, must be a crackpot.

Only on one thing in fighting the virus do all

doctors agree: Rest. Outside of that, personal opinion rules, and every advice and prescription is based on personal deductions. Unfortunately, one has been as good as the other.

No one really knows why some people don't catch colds at all. Year in and year out, some people don't catch colds and seem to have permanent immunity—they don't even catch mild colds. In the coldest weather most of these people don't wear topcoats because they are cumbersome and weighty. Also it seems in a real life-and-death crisis, not related to illness, one becomes immune no matter how prone to catching a cold one has been during the course of his lifetime.

We have heard of airline crashes on a snow-covered plain or mountain. Among the survivors, frost-bite is frequently reported, but rarely a case of influenza or a common cold.

I met an Armenian from Soviet Armenia before the Soviet Union dismantled. Prior to the earthquake in that region, he had acquired an exit permit to visit his relatives in Iran. He was among a number of people on the first floor of a government apartment building when the quake came.

Those on the first floor dashed for the basement just before the total collapse of the building. For twelve days they were trapped in the basement. They had food and candles, because a section of the basement was either a food store or food storage house of some sort for the residents of the building.

The burly, ruddy-faced Armenian whom I met in the apartment of one of his relatives in Tehran was not inclined toward exchange of dialogue or conversation. Brought up in a society where reticence was elemental to survival, he mostly shook his head or nodded assent, or offered short comments. Glasnost evidently did not seem yet to have put any noticeable impression on him. Or, perhaps the earthquake was an experience he did not want to talk about—just like war veterans are reluctant to talk about their war memories.

I gathered from his relatives that for twelve days he, along with the others trapped in the basement, had had enough to eat. They were cold, with only the flame of a single candle, lit one after another, to keep their fingers warm and functioning.

I asked the man, "Did any of you have a cold or influenza when you were rescued?"

The man was peeling a cucumber. Pausing, and slightly amused, he placed a peeled skin carefully on a platter, and without looking up, replied, "When you are faced with death, you don't catch cold."

He didn't say anything more and I didn't question him further, because I felt I was straining him.

No thorough and conclusive research has been made as to why we catch colds at all. After centuries of stereotyped thinking we have to drop off trying to find the cause outside of ourselves. This notion of being "caught in a rain without an umbrella," or "having no hat on while walking on the streets in a cold autumn wind" and so on must be discarded as the reasons for catching cold. People catch cold and go on to the flu stage right in the heat of the summer.

Most summer colds come from car air-conditioners, which like nasal passages provide a suitable place for the virus to sustain itself. The evaporator, the cold surface of the coil on which the air inside the car passes and delivers its heat, is always moist with condensation. It is cool and dark there and moisture mixed with street dust drips from the coil surfaces.

Remember, the virus does not need human blood to survive. It thrives in moisture and dust. When the air-conditioner is off and you start it after several hours, an unhealthy, hot and vapid humid air blasts out of the outlets first before gradually cooling. This indicates the presence of humidity. All it takes is one with a cold to sneeze in a new car and the aerosol droplets spewed out find a nice cool humid home on the evaporator-coil surface of the air conditioner.

All cars, old and new, provide plenty of healthy and vigorous viruses for the breathing organs of the passengers who ride in air-conditioned cars. The same goes for buses, trains and planes.

But why do only a few isolated cases catch cold from this lively and permanent source during the whole summer? Why so much exposure and so little infection? Why no epidemic? Why, when a member of the family catches a summer cold, the rest of the family members do not catch it? Or if they do, it is a rare thing. Why no person-to-person transmission during summer months?

I think that as the visitor from Soviet Armenia indirectly put it, ones state of mind has a lot to do with it. Summer is a time of travel, vacations, picnics, outdoors, barbecues, no schools, well-lit lawns and drunken guffaws heard from distant homes in all the neighborhoods in any country. If you or your next door neighbor is giving a party outside, you too contribute to the jubilation and your laughter is heard by others in the neighborhood.

Summer is fiesta worldwide and when it ends, the bright jubilant smiles on faces are not quite there anymore, heartfully and exhiliaratingly. There is a let-down, a subtle one, at the end of each summer, and the human mind collectively experiences mild depression not quite consciously felt.

The virus comes, confident, not because the autumn has arrived, but because the summer has ended. The fiesta is over. You have a sense of having put one section of the good life behind you, and it may or may never come again. There are only worries and hard work on ahead, particularly for the students. With the advent of a grey winter the virus overcomes, and that is my personal opinion based on observation and guesswork.

The sixteenth century poet, William Cowper, must have agreed with me when he wrote:

> O'Winter! ruler of the inverted year
> Thy scattered hair with sleet like ashes filled
> Thy breath congealed upon thy lips, thy cheeks
> Fringed with a beard made white with other
>   snows
> than those of age . . .

What you read above fully supports my point of view and "white with other snows than those of age" carries weight and meaning in the direction of wintertime gloom, escapable only when you have a home in Florida or Palm Springs to live in until springtime.

The green is gone and the trees look like wood sticking out of earth scorched by the cold. And you have caught the cold. If you have done nothing to prevent it, you soon are in the advanced stages of the cold. Your nose is plugged and every time you blow it you hear a horn-like noise, and your brain seems to be coming out in liquid form.

I suggest that in the advanced stages of the cold you have the nose wash, quick, with the vitamin C solution. I repeat. Crush a 500 mg tablet in a normal drinking glass. Add water until it is a quarter-full. Stir, draw it up from your cupped hand into your nostrils and nasal passages three or four times, and get it all out so you can breathe—through the nose, not the mouth.

When your breathing becomes easy, you can rest better. This works like an anti-depressant. You sense the early signs of recovery, and this helps increase your resistance.

Forego the gamma globulin shot. Because, at an advanced stage of the cold, you weaken the full-blooming virus to a level it becomes similar to a vaccine, but after considerable suffering.

You want to get rid of the cold as fast as you can, you want to go to work, and you want to go on with life. Get an intravenous 500 CC injection of vitamin C and see what will happen. Immediately after the shot the flow from the nose increases, and if you cough, you will cough with force and with more discharge. For a couple of hours it will seem like you have become worse. The nose drips like a leaking faucet. It seems you have sunk further and deeper in the wretchedness of the illness. To some this may appear to be a mistake, but it is not. You are already getting well much sooner than you anticipated. The mucus discharge which would normally take two to three days is being done within two to three hours. The virus is being kicked out, washed out, and the disease is passing its peak, quick.

There is a fruit in Iran and I don't know of it being available in the U.S. It is called sweet-lemon and it is very good for you while you are having a cold. Sweet lemon is a citrus fruit, very sweet in taste and good for all illnesses except di-arrhea. It is rich with vitamin C.

Eating this fruit is refreshing, and you can eat a basket-full. When taking an antibiotic, it is great stuff for filtering out the toxins that the an-tibiotic produces in your blood. It has a greater reputation of being a medical fruit than an enjoy-ment fruit, and if fruits were allowed to be im-ported to the U.S., I would have telexed my of-fice to airfreight two crates for you, Tammy. Perhaps contact between us would be made fi-nally through sweet lemons.

Why don't you call? Why the silence? Are you set on being a lost friend forever? Are you really down with a cold? Have you, like me, mar-ried again, have you remarried your ex-husband, are you on a secret honeymoon somewhere in Europe or Florida, and your secretary is protect-ing your secret? Or is she protecting your rest? If the latter is the case, rest while I write.

Do nothing more than rest. You may be bored with resting but try to like it. Enjoy the perfect idleness, watch the ceiling if you are not sleeping. Let your thoughts float. That is the best state of mind when you are down with a cold.

The theory of quick response is conductive to your being up on your feet when fighting a cold, and not losing a day's work. But when you succumb to a cold, stay down. Lay down to rest in an absolute sense. Don't pick up a magazine or a book to read. Don't even watch television. A heart-rending drama or watching news broadcasts with all its shock and excitement puts your mind, the very center of your existence, into active service. Avoid that.

Experiment with yourself if you want and see what absolute rest means. When you are resting and your mind is not active on any particular subject or idea, and you are not having a brainstorm—the cold won't seem to be with you. But take a newspaper and read, and soon a sneeze or two comes, and you have to reach for the tissue box. Stop reading and you will be back in the dry state. Repeat again and the same thing happens. There is a direct relationship between the idleness of the mind and the drip, as sure as the unfaltering law of gravity.

Don't do the company's work while you're in bed with a cold, even if it is merely reading a report or making sketches for a design. You won't serve the company's cause by doing beyond the call of duty work and causing the extension of your illness. Just rest. Let a tranquilizer help you if you are bored and want to do something. Keep yourself in a state of not wanting to do anything as long as you can. When you are fit for work, you will know it.

Don't dash to work out of eagerness, or go early with the telltale signs of the cold—the sore edges of your nostrils and the upper lip only prove to the boss you were not loafing. But the boss passing good judgment on you doesn't speed your good riddance of the cold.

Remember, as long as you sneeze when out of bed several times a day, you are still flu-ridden and you can infect your associates as well as the family, and nothing can be done about it as long as the method I've shared with you is not practiced by all.

Under the circumstances give your associates the chance of getting infected from other sources rather than from you. At the same time keep in mind that if your job needs you badly, and you feel that you must attend to something important, by all means go to work and don't mind how many people you will flatten with the residue of your cold. If your associates don't get it from you, they will get it from others. Thus, you will not do them harm if out of no choice you infect a few. Only in this regard, try to maintain an ethical balance.

While lying in bed with a cold, resting, having nothing to do, being away from the commotion and stresses of daily life, and being the recipient of special care and attention of your spouse, things sometimes steer off course. A problem may arise that brings a setback. A strong desire for the ultimate in togetherness may surface and if things happen, in whatever stage of the cold you are in, you will get worse. You have to be with the virus for a couple more days. But what is two or three days in a lifetime?

To my mind comes the refrains of an old song the frat-boys sang at their drunken beer parties:

"I can't give you anything but love, baby..."

I don't remember the remaining lines, Tammy. My head is full of fragments of songs I heard when we were together in a singing crowd. You sung in harmony with others, but I listened. The tunes of the ballads of love from the twenties with their sweet, timeless innocence are all in my head, but not quite the lyrics. Here is one:

"Saturday night...
I wait for you, honey,
at half past eight."

And so, I wait.

Chapter IV

If during the course of a cold you feel well rested and your flame is around catering, and you are in the mood, why not? Threats of any kind would not be imposed on the establishment nor would it cause humanity any harm. Let the virus revel in triumph for a day or two. It may even be medically justified if the temptation endures and keeps interfering with your sleep.

In regard to your immediate family, insist on the exercise of the method even if they think you are a lunatic. That's what my wife thought I was at the beginning. If I force-dropped vitamin C solution in our child's nose, it had to be done when she was not around. Her response to my confession always came with the accusation that my treatment of the child would shame a fiend.

But her anger always subsided after she saw the quick improvement of the child's condition. Now she is a practitioner of the method herself. My ninety-one-year-old mother, with quick injections of vitamin C and gamma globulin shots, hasn't been bothered with a cold for several years.

At the onset, I repeat, the VC wash gives you time till you reach someone who could give you the injections. For old people the VC wash is not mandatory if the wash, with its temporal discomfort, is too much for the old person.

When feeling not clean, by all means, take a bath. But not the type that would strain you. Don't sit in a hot tub for a half-hour. Don't shower with very hot water so your body sweats afterward to get rid of the excess heat. That is strain.

Take a short shower with lukewarm water and shampoo your hair, too, if you have an electric hair-dryer. Make your hair absolute dry after washing. Make sure your room is warm. Put on fresh, dry underwear and pajamas, go to bed, and cover yourself to the chin. Put on a home headwear of any kind if you have it, but take it off as soon as you feel your head is about to sweat.

Taking a shower as described makes your skin breathe and on the whole makes you feel good. Taking a bath during a cold is good, provided you don't go around doing house-chores.

Now, as I said before, after the treatment, don't eat or drink anything cold. Eat only nutritious foods.

For anyone recovering from a cold, and for those practitioners of the method who have stopped the cold at the onset, this instruction has one flaw: Because you don't have the feeling you had a bout with the cold, rarely will you remember to take the proper care. Somebody shoves a drink into your hand with ice, and you take a couple of gulps before remembering your condition. You take an apple out of the refrigerator and unknowingly start biting. Unless you are one of those health fanatics, who, in good health, can look at a cold apple for a half-hour because the chill in it is bad for teeth, you are bound to make the mistake of eating the cold apple, or you will finish your drink and soon feel a wrinkly feeling at the base of your throat.

With short coughs you keep clearing your throat, but the coarse, uneven sensation doesn't go away. To correct that feeling you drink something warm, a hot tea or coffee, but the same, ill-omened sensation remains. The virus, with a changed structure and personality, has come to new hospitable territory, the upper respiratory tract and eventually the lower one: your lungs.

You have to act fast again, otherwise your lungs will become congested, and might churn out phlegm for the rest of the winter. This would be more at the beginning and less later on, but it will take you a long time to be rid of it.

You must have the right antibiotic ready in the medicine cabinet. Ampicillin of 500 mg strength would do well. Before you reach your doctor, begin taking the antibiotics, one capsule every eight hours. Also take an expectorant before your lungs become phlegmatic, otherwise, until warm weather comes, you will go around bringing up phlegm with a sudden short cough in the most unexpected place or situation. Sometimes you may be forced to drop it on the side-walk when no one is looking.

But, of course, you wouldn't do a thing like that. You are different, Tammy. You belong to a worldwide sect called the beautiful people in your country. That makes you special. The beautiful are the ones different, not the rich.

Now you are rich and no doubt still beauti-ful—I hope you remain that way ever—but be-ware that the all-knowing God at times plays rough games with his chosen children. Give a mind to this: the great Iranian painter Kamalel-molk became blind in old age, Beethoven became deaf, and the late billionaire Paul Getty got dys-pepsia. Could calamities so devastatingly ironic be holy jokes? Or, could we surmise that all are acts of holy balance? God gives, God takes. One really can't figure these things out without a sense of religiousness. Why is it that those so lav-ishly blessed with talent die early? They expire, because in the time of their lives they have to burn bright. Longevity is not luck; talent is.

It remains in the universal order of things that when God takes, ample compensation already has been given. Beethoven's "Symphony Number Nine" is the closest thing to God singing music to his children. What if the chosen source were stars in heaven, becoming comets while they sang it together? Of what importance that at the end of a shiny trail, however short, is extinction?

So what if with equal irony, you being now a successful designer of fashion end up in old age in rags, not of pecuniary reason, but by an aberration of concepts and ideas? Am I putting you in the category of those mentioned so that a likely loss of reasoning may counterbalance your success?

Not at all. Let's say I am giving you the scare just because you haven't returned my call. The phone in my room is unreasonably silent.

When you are suffering with a cough, you need to lie down for days, and have warm liquid and hot food, but you can't bring yourself to the level of the eat-and-do-nothing stage. That can't be done. You must have an antibiotic, but you can't have it. You have to go do a doctor to get a prescription, then to the pharmacist in your drugstore. How long a lapse of time? At least two days, more if you are afflicted on a weekend.

In the news we read about important people who recently have died of pneumonia, or we read about movie stars, now recuperating from respiratory afflictions. They are examples, regardless of their fame. They represent the nearly ten thousand people who die every year because of cold-related illnesses in the U.S. alone, and their condition doesn't make news. The majority perhaps are heavy smokers with health dimmed by alcohol or advanced age.

But when stricken, first the uncaring attitude of yesteryear comes into play and forces people to ignore it initially. Precious hours are lost doing just about nothing. Just rest and you will be all right is the common thinking. With the severity of the illness becoming clear, they finally go to a doctor. Afterward either they come home, or they go to a hospital. Later, they will recuperate after the illness at home, if they are lucky.

Now what if these people had taken a dose of antibiotics according to their own judgment at the earliest sign of having a little discomfort in the lungs, before reaching a doctor to check the sound of the respiration with a stethoscope? Antibiotics don't kill anybody if taken without a doctor's prescription, and if you are allergic to a certain brand, you know it before the doctor. And one antibiotic pill taken on the first day is worth ten taken three days later. The same goes with cortisone pills of 0.5 mg strength, which, according to personal judgment, could also be taken.

The doctor may advise you not to take what you are taking, or give you a different medicine, but whatever kind of antibiotic you take on your own at the onset is the most effective and undeniably the best first-aid you can get. And first-aid doesn't seem to exist, outside of the aspirin-family for the patient with an oncoming severe influenza, and perhaps pneumonia later, or some bad after-effects later still.

Why are a few capsules of antibiotics denied over-the-counter? A healthy person is unable to get them, but when stricken, and after the magnitude of the illness becomes grave, at least fifty ampules of gentomycin are added to the patient's injection schedule to fight the flagrant infection in the lungs.

Why is it justified that a person, for first-aid, should sit and pray and wait for the night to pass for an early visit to a doctor the next day and not be able to do anything for himself? Why should he not have a good fighting chance on his own before reaching a doctor?

So by all means every year refurbish your medicine cabinet by whatever forbidden means possible for your own quick, personal no-waiting-for-the-doctor response.

In every respect, time lapse is the virus' best ally. Why do you think that the heads of states never cancel a trip or visit? Why don't you ever hear that President Clinton is down with a cold resting in the White House for a few days?

The same thing goes for all heads of state all over the globe. Quick response is available to them through their personal physicians, who are members of their staff. They push a button and their doctor comes. You, too, should push a button in your head to become your own doctor when the early symptoms come. It is not the doctor who quickly cures a president's cold, it is the striking back quickly that cures.

Catching cold, year after year, has given you enough experience to make you a first-rate doctor for yourself in this particular field. Not falling in the clutches of a cold to an extent that would disrupt your work should not remain a luxury for the VIPs only. You just need to know how to cure a common cold at the onset fast, without after-effects.

Taking antibiotics as preventive medicine for infection is not without precedent. When a patient undergoes surgery in a hospital, antibiotics are given to prevent infection. Why doesn't the same concept hold good for a pair of lungs about to be congested with pathogenic agents, or in a simple word—pus? Should this condition be taken lightly because it is not accompanied with fever, and it is expected that you can live with it for a period of time which sometimes can be the whole winter?

It is better to take antibiotics before your lungs get infected. Take plenty of vitamin C in the form of sherbet, 1500 mg twice a day. Use three tablets of this vitamin, crush them into powder form, add tap water and sugar in a glass, stir and drink it.

It is a very tasteful drink, and you won't mind having it even for several days more after you are quite well. Drink this when you are likely to have a drink of some sort. Don't allow yourself to think that it should be after meals, during or before. Your next meal may be two hours away. Drink it when you know you can absorb it quickly and not necessarily at any set time. A simple thirst for water could justify it.

You are lucky if your lot after a cold is a wet cough, which eventually phases out and does not hamper your sleep. With a dry cough you suffer more because you can't sleep at night. Every night, without relief in sight, is a long night's journey into morning. When the sweet doze-off comes, you are suddenly jolted into a whitish awakeness by a cough so violent that it shakes your being down to every nerve-root. In desperation you might swallow a cough-depressant or you may put a cough drop into your cheek and close your eyes, only to have the violent cough come again after you fall into a brief sleep. Three or four times this happens, and then sleep and you become total strangers for the rest of the night.

During the day you repeatedly fall into fits of coughing, sometimes for no understandable reason, and sometimes when you whiff in a wisp of cigarette smoke passing under your nose, perfume, lotion, sprays, exhaust fumes, pollen, dust—anything, not necessarily with an odor. This condition is unlikely to phase itself out during the winter and usually happens to people who take up their drinking habit too soon after a cold.

Alcohol is the worst thing, at the onset, during the course of a cold, and soon after. It makes your lungs temporarily allergic to virtually everything. When in such a condition, avoid cough drops or antihistamines.

Take the ultimate course. Don't waste a lot of time going through chest x-rays, blood tests and so on, then be told that nothing is wrong, and that your condition is caused only by post-nasal drip! If you think that is the right diagnosis, wash your nasal passages with salt water, and gargle with the rest of it in the glass.

When you cannot sleep at night because of the cough, which you know is the residue of a bout with a cold, no matter how long ago. And during the day when you breathe in air and exhalation tends to be in the form of a cough, and the repeated fits of hernia-hurting coughs come more than you can tolerate; take the ultimate solution.

If you don't have stomach ulcers, don't waste time. Take cortisone pills of 0.5 mg strength along with an antibiotic three times a day. Ampicillin will do—capsules of 500 mg once every eight hours. You will get rid of the cough within the first day of the take.

You sleep a drug-free sleep, because you owe yourself so much sleep that you don't need pills to induce it. Continue this treatment for ten days, but taper off the dosage of the cortisone pills from the fifth day on until it becomes almost nil on the tenth day. By then you will be totally free from the black cough which ruined your sleep and brought nocturnal despair for you and your family.

Remember also something else. Even to healthy people, the bloating of the stomach at night with raw fruit, beans, salad, milk, ice cream or any dairy products like yogurt, cheese or starchy food, aggravates a dry cough badly and could bring night coughs.

Forego even the supposedly curative warm glass of milk and aspirin before bedtime. Those mentioned are all gas-producing food items which make you belch (according to your choice, either loud or quietly), and just because you cannot do that while lying down, your throat tickles as part of a nervous response to a needed release that cannot take place. You wake up, sitting in bed coughing violently and glaring in the dark. Sometimes gas purges through between coughs. Diet plays a big role here.

Try to sleep on a lean, near hungry stomach all year round if you have problems coughing at night. That helps your quick recovery from a persistent cold-cough also.

Some people, for good measure, drink several cups of hot tea with half of a lemon squeezed in it, thinking that it warms their throat and passes vitamin C over the aggravated tissues of the throat and also provides an abundant supply of vitamin C to the body. This is the worst thing you can do. This even brings coughs to healthy people because of a sour stomach. Forego even the vitamin C sherbet when you have a dry cough. A sour stomach, without you even feeling it, makes the throat tickle and you cough.

Here's another point to consider. When you are well, always let the tasty dressing remain in the bowl after you finish your salad. Don't drink it.

And, of course, you know that too much coffee gives you a nervous stomach and that make you cough also. If you are not a smoker and you don't want unjustified coughs, play fair with your stomach.

Obviously, there are times when you just can't do that. You just can't play fair because over-filling your stomach at a good dinner party is unavoidable.

Or, you let yourself become too hungry, and you sit at the dinner table and you eat. You eat long after you had enough because your mind, due to its pre-set conditioning having received so many hungry signals, cannot tune itself with the eating race. You eat until your stomach literally has no more room or space. For lack of space you don't eat anymore and not because you are no longer hungry. That is gluttony, one of the Seven Deadly Sins. But it is not too grave a sin if you do it only once in a while.

When bedtime comes and you are overfilled, pump the gas out of your stomach by kicking one foot at a time up in the air like a soccer player. Do this exercise for fifteen minutes, not necessarily continuously, rest in between. After a while gas starts purging upward sporadically, but in an amount that eventually could fill a bicycle tube. Aside from the advantage of relieving your stomach to make you sleep better, this exercise, if done every night for years, not necessarily for the stomach, is bound to give you the build of a flamenco dancer regardless of your age. All you will be needing then, Tammy, would be a pair of castanets.

Suddenly I recollect your repeated smiles the first time I tried to teach you backgammon—a word so unknown those days in the english-speaking world that one probingly could have guessed backgammon to be the name of a tropicla tree.

And I recall trying to learn this song from you once when we were on a picnic. I may keep searching for its meaning, forever.

> Chicori chic chola chola
> Chicori chic in a vananeka
> Chicori chic chola cholaaa . . .
> Chicori chic is me.

But what greater meaning can there be that you and I once sang it, and our voices mixed, and we stopped to laugh at my clumsiness in learning those idiotically charming words?

One with a big girth, in a year with the soccer-kick exercise, may run out of notch-holes on the trouser's belt. In two, the need may arise to purchase a new belt and trousers altogether.

You can pump your stomach by kicking up a bended knee. This keeps your center of gravity nearer to where it was before, reducing the risk

❧

of falling or gyrating out of balance. Rhythmi-
cally, with each thigh, give a jolt to your stomach. Do this, even if you are already too big to
let fly a soccer kick. Start it off so. Don't risk a
fall if you are big and middle-aged. Of course
stationary bicycling in front of television would
do the same thing for you.

Chapter V

So this is it, Tammy. This is all I know about how not to catch a cold.

Throughout the years, when down with a bad cold—mine always became the worst because I never rested until I literally buckled—I was so miserable that I tried every means to be free of it. Once, several years ago, I heard over Israeli radio that when hot air is blasted into the nose the virus in the passage dies because of the intolerable high temperature and you become free of the cold. That, I proved to myself to be pure nonsense.

During my spare time before the season, I built myself a small electrical warm-air furnace with a fan. I taped it to my nose with two flexible tubes the size of my nostrils. When I caught the cold, I blasted in the hot air, keeping my mouth open to regulate breathing. Sure enough, it evaporated the moistness. Then, after about one hour of applying the heat, I removed the tubes. I was in a dry state for a while, only for a while. Then gradually the nose started delivering. Before long, good as ever.

Once the virus bug bites, overheating may make the bug listless but never causes it to loosen its clutch. This I proved to myself before I came to a happy, emphatic conclusion with my own method.

Keep also in mind that some medical researchers argue that when you inoculate yourself with gamma globulin you hamper your body's immune system. If this is true, why is gamma globulin being manufactured? Two cc of gamma globulin once a year is not going to hinder the body's immune system. If it increases your body's resistance to a number of viral infections during winter why not use it? Ten gamma globulin ampules may be required for some imaginary illness that may come your way in the future, they argue. Those prone to such thinking are not practical thinkers, but if it is good for you now, why not use it? The doctors can take care of bigger, more complicated illnesses if it is your lot to suffer them in some distant future.

I know of people who proudly won't take an aspirin for a headache, thinking they are disciplining their body, making it fit to stand up on its own to ailments without the aid of pills. These people are not disciplining anything. They only extend their suffering as long as a caveman did back in the Stone Age.

When ill, take a pill. Take ample dosages of whatever medicine is good for you to fight the onrush of an ailment or a disease. Don't go for that let-the-body-carry-on-its-own-fight stuff. That's foolishness at its peak.

We are now reaching the apex of the pyramid, Tammy, the final say on the subject of how not to catch a cold.

If I had said this all to you in a single page letter you likely would not have believed me. Please believe me, especially now, after all the work I have done. This is a benediction.

It has been five years since I have had injections of vitamin C or gamma globulin. Nor have I snorted up into my nose any vitamin C solution. I haven't needed to, because in the last five years I have not come down with a cold.

I don't know what has taken place. I don't know the chemical side of it. I don't know anything about chromosomes, split-genes, DNA, and much less do I know about microbiology or virology and all other aspects of medical science. All I know is that I just don't catch colds anymore. I have come upon a mine of gold without looking for it.

In the first five years, with the aid of those self-tested treatments, I thought I would be free of severe bouts with cold forever, but not without the exercise of the method. Now I am free of all of them without the need whatsoever for any treatment. There are only days in autumn that I use my handkerchief too often, without knowing whether the cause is hay fever, an allergy, or an invading cold. If the latter is the case, the invasion does not get anywhere. It passes. For safe measure I drink a glass or two a day of vitamin C sherbet.

What has happened?

Is it all due to a new state of mind as the old Armenian implied? Have I licked the problem of catching cold because I am always prepared for a bout? Have I developed an icy, lethal stare when I enter the ring with the virus? Does the virus fear me? Does it know I am the victor always in the first round? Does the virus have a mind? Can it think twice? Does it know whom to avoid and whom to attack? Or is it all chemical?

Have I slowly built up in myself a lifelong immunity by the method? Or is it a combination— mental and chemical both? An invincible mental state would not be achieved without catching the cold, then knowing you could lick it in a single afternoon.

Aiding the body massively to fight an incipient cold is all a different story than having flu shots on time. I have seen a few cases of the kind of cold that people come down with having had flu shots. The symptoms are all there; all that of a full-fledged cold requiring rest and some medication. Only the young can pass through it uncaringly. The nose drips, eyes water and there are sneezes. This sense of security that the condition will not worsen, will not plummet into pneumonia, bone aches, fever, lung or ear infection is all very fine.

If you can't accept my method, by all means have flu shots. But if you want not to catch a cold at all, year after year, go with what I prescribe. Permeate your mind with this sense of invincibility, this sense of quiet security that you have life-long immunity and you don't need to fortify yourself with shots of any kind when you are well and walking. And don't go with this night-nurse and day-nurse stuff, and don't swallow all this slush advertised on television that with a spoonful you pass off into a deep, dreamlike sleep without flip-flops, no toss and turns, through the night, when you are down with a cold.

Let's go back to the basics.

For a good night's rest you need a clear and clean breathing passage. So wash the nose amply with vitamin C solution, get all the crud out, dislodge it completely.

Believe me, it is worth the bearing of a few seconds of discomfort. The benefits are manyfold when it makes your breathing through the night so much freer and easier, with none of that unnatural snoring and wheezing that causes repeated waking up by the reverberation of the noises of your own making in your head. When you can breathe naturally and easily through the nose, sleep comes easily, and in long duration with a couple of micro-coated aspirin or better with a sleeping pill.

And don't forget the vitamin C shot and the gamma globulin shot the next day, both in quick succession. The two shots, when they mix in blood, make a special kind of chemistry that knocks the virus out in a short spell, and makes the symptoms of a cold almost nonexistent.

I cannot tell you anything about the whys of the process that take place that cause such quick beneficial results. Let those who want to do the research. The problem is solved for me in the best possible way at this stage of my life.

It was good writing you this long letter, Tammy.

So preoccupied I was with your thought, never for a moment had I the desire to go down and sit in the hotel lobby and ogle. The spacious bar below with the stained glass and soft lights and scented air flowing out its arched doorway seemed also very inviting. But I didn't go there either, not even for a beer. I wrote this letter to you cold sober.

Now, shortly I am flying to Europe to loiter there for a couple of weeks and then to Iran, which to you was and perhaps still is, as always, Persia. I never forget how your eyes glowed with light whenever the historical name of Iran was mentioned. You never used the name Iran when we were students because Persia rang romantic bells in your ears. It made you think of flying carpets, handsome sheiks and harem houris, and just because I came from there you thought also that I was an authentic specimen right out of the pages of *The Thousand and One Nights.* That was youth, Tammy.

Your memory is the memory of my youth itself with all its luminous moments now frozen in the frame of time, blessing this old friend with a possession so cherishable that it brims me with inexhaustible exuberance when I look back on it.

❦

The memories of you and the world in which you live have not become yet shades and shadows. They are there, clear and fresh, as if all belonging only to yesterday.

I don't feel snubbed that you didn't call me. All I hope is that you never catch cold again. I hope you will call me someday.

In the meantime, don't go from one cold on to the next. You don't have to. Read my letter again and carry on with the fight. And be as good as you always were.

I will mail this letter from Tehran after I have it typed.

H.D.

Epilogue

In the annals of medicine, there is a world outside medical schools—not as rich in knowledge, but as old as mankind—its benefits never officially acknowledged, but here with us, unheralded, ridding us of many tenacious undetectable ailments.

Ever since I can remember, I have heard of one-prescription doctors, the general practitioner to whom you don't have to go twice for the same sickness. The medicine and dosage patently the same, the cure with certain doctors comes quickly. What could this be attributed to, except that the fast-curing doctors, without themselves knowing, treat patients with a touch of healing power. If I am correct, how vastly complex and expansive are the arenas of treatment and curing, and how beneficial, sometimes, could be the medical advice passed from one person to the other.

Beginning about four years ago, my eyes took on the habit of watering—not profusely, but noticeably. When I had a brief laugh, I had to take my glasses off and wipe the water that would roll down like tears if I didn't. If I watched a sad drama on television, I had to have a handkerchief ready in hand. And if I made a speech addressing the personnel and the workforce of the factory, I often overwhelmed myself with my own words and had to pause to regain emotional control. Eventually, I came to the sad conclusion that because of overactive moisturing glands somewhere in my eyes, I was gradually becoming lugubrious. The uncalled-for tears brought along the unwanted sadness.

The ophthalmologists I went to, assured me the fine drainage canals in the lower corner of the eyes were open and functioning. They all sent me home with various harmless eyedrops, not wanting to hurt my feelings with the unmentionable diagnosis!

Then came the time I had guests in Tehran from the United Arab Emirates, one being an architect working in Dubai. We gathered in a countryside home, sitting around a fireplace. Jokes were flying and there were many laughs, which made me take my glasses off repeatedly to prepare my eyes with my handkerchief for the next round of laughs. The talk drifted onto the subject of my book. A discussion started about the vitamin C wash of the nasal passage. The distinguished architect from Dubai concurred with me on this. Along the line of thought that one would get used to any temporary discomfort, he recommended drops of purified, fresh onion juice in the eyes three times a week for keeping the eyes in absolutely perfect health. Even for me, this was jolting, but his friends seemed to know. Evidently he practiced what he preached. I looked in the man's eyes and for the first time I noticed the remarkable sheen. The eyes looked so much younger than the man; did not have the slightest extra moisture in them; were well focused, and swiftly moved. As we talked, I noticed the eyes darted, rather than rolled, towards the objects of sight, and covered larger vistas of vision without the craning of neck or shoulders.

It took me three months to muster up enough courage to drop onion juice in my eyes. When I did, I knew I would never do it again, but the evening of that particular day I went to a dinner party. Never before had I felt so confident and never before can I remember being so alert and whole. My eyes, naturally small, felt so much larger than before. I felt great. I walked erect and tall, as if there were a halo of happiness around my head.

The well-being of my eyes lasted two days, but I was not to part with the good feeling. For years, I had heard that onions are rich with vitamin C. So there! The connection! I was to walk on my own familiar grounds.

As I write these words, it has been three months now that I have kept a medicine bottle of potent and filtered vitamin C solution in the refrigerator. From it, each night before sleep I take the eyedropper out and literally wash my eyes with ample drops. My eyes may never feel as resplendent as the night I went to that dinner party, but never have they watered intolerably, either. Thanks to a friend, and a man to be remembered: Amar Chawla of Dubai.

H. Dehesh

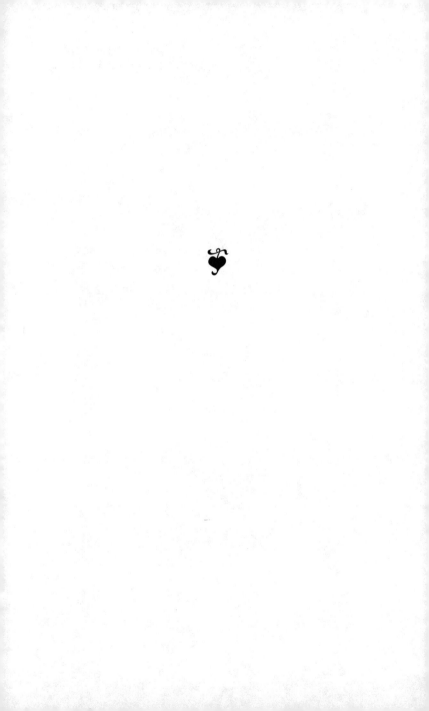